CHRONIC PAIN RELIEF:
12 NON-MEDICAL APPROACHES
(REVISED)

DAVID ABBEY, PH.D.

Acknowledgments

While this book is about non-medical approaches to the relief of chronic pain I must acknowledge the efforts of the various medical and other specialists who deal with their patients' distress. Day after day they are confronted with a reality which they cannot experience directly and which is frustrating, demoralizing and sometimes life-threatening for their patients.

In my own clinical practice I have encountered people of incredible emotional and spiritual strength who have tolerated years of agony. Their stories have been among the prompts to write this book.

Finally, there are the families of the chronic pain patient. As a family therapist I have seen the chaos and confusion which can result as patience wears thin, helplessness sets in, and anger replaces love and care. In many cases wives, mothers and children are able to rise above these; in other cases, families and couples dissolve. I salute those who "stay the course" and offer support and encouragement and who continue to believe that with work (and perhaps faith) some relief can be found.

Table of Contents

About the Author (and *his* pain)

David Abbey is a Registered Psychologist with over 45 years of experience as a clinician. His focus for many years has been on the problems which his clients (and frequently their families) have in dealing with chronic pain. For several decades David suffered with extreme leg and back pain and he went the rounds of practitioners looking for help.

At one time or another he has been a patient of: a general practitioner; an orthopedic surgeon; a physiotherapist; a chiropractor; a kinesiologist; a massage therapist and a Doctor of Traditional Chinese Medicine. He also studied and tried a wide variety of healing approaches such as: reflexology; Rolfing; meditation, and hypnosis. At one point, a young man who had recently graduated from a course in Applied Kinesiology put together a set of simple stretches and bends that apparently "cured" the problem for several years.

Unhappily, he has not lived "happily ever after". The pain returned and in 2014 following an MRI it became apparent that there was an underlying condition called "spinal stenosis" – a narrowing of the spinal canal which results in compression of the nerves leading to the low back and legs. Next to be considered is a course of treatment involving nerve blocks and possibly surgery. "We can but hope."

While waiting, David continues to use many of the techniques described in this book. He's happy to share them with you, the reader.

David lives in Guelph, Ontario, Canada with his wife Susan who is a marriage and family therapist (see her website, www.dafoe-abbey.com !). Between them they have six children, seven grand-children and an active counseling and coaching practice in Guelph, Ontario.

BUT:

> David's story is not your story. His back is not your back; and what has worked for him to provide relief may not work for you.

SO:

> Use this book as a collection of descriptions of what some people have found helpful in their lives. If one or more of the approaches seems interesting and you want to try it (them) <u>talk it over with your health care practitioner(s)</u>.

> Your physician knows far more about the body (and in particular about your body) than most other professionals and should be involved in any changes you are considering.

> Don't quit any treatment or drugs which may have been prescribed for you without talking it over with the people who have been caring for you.

AND:

> Approach this book, the exercises and the examples with a sense of curiosity. Wonder whether, or how, or why the various approaches work. Then plunge in and experience the results. Behave like an explorer – always wondering what's around the next bend; observing; maybe taking notes and always curious.

Who is this book for?

Let me start by saying that all of the techniques described in this book could, at some time or another, be useful to anyone experiencing pain. However, I wrote it with a particular group of people in mind:

those who have been experiencing chronic pain and for whom the usual (traditional) approaches do not appear to be working as well as they could.

Let me give you three examples:

(1)Judy has had surgery on both wrists for Carpal Tunnel Syndrome. The operations were both successful. The pressure on the nerves was reduced; the incisions healed, and she engaged in the post-op exercises as prescribed.

That was 3 years ago. To-day, she complains of what she calls "incredible, continuous burning" in her wrists – but sometimes, she says, "the feeling is like an ice-pick jabbing between the bones in her wrist".

The pain-killers which have been prescribed leave her dizzy and unable to attend to the details of her work.

(2)Franz was hit by a car as he crossed the street near his home. He was thrown several feet and landed on his shoulder with a broken collar-bone, and a fractured forearm and a crushed hand.

Three surgeries to repair the nerves in his hand have given him some movement in his fingers which had been paralyzed and a continuous "screaming" pain that shoots up and down his arm. Damp and cold weather make the pain worse and the only real relief he experiences comes from illegal drugs.

(3)Beatrice frequently experiences rectal cramps which leave her exhausted and in tears from the pain. Various diets, medication and bed-rest have not helped and she suffers almost daily from this disorder.

So, these are three cases from among many similar - and often heart-breaking - clients. What they have in common is that despite the dedicated care given to them by their primary care specialists they still hurt.

The treatment which has been provided is likely the best that can be given. But in many cases pain seems to have a life and a mind of its own. It simply doesn't go away, or does go away and then reappears in the same place or somewhere else in the body.

This book was written so that if you happen to be someone who doesn't seem to respond to treatment in the expected way, you might find another approach to experiment with.

Not many of the methods described in this book will help if the pain you experience has lasted for about 3 minutes and is from a stubbed toe. But if the pain is still there 3 or 6 months later and X-rays and ultrasound say, "nothing is wrong", then maybe something here will be helpful.

Why is Pain such a Problem?

Saul has had chronic pain in his shoulder for more than a year. He remembers hearing a "pop" when he was playing catch with his son and after a few days of discomfort he went for massage.

The massage helped a great deal but he was still left with a nagging jolt every time he lifted his arm up to shoulder height. In fact, the pain has been getting worse but when Saul tries to describe it he sometimes uses the word "jolt"; at other times he uses words such as: stabbing; piercing, and even tearing.

The sensation is sometimes heat and sometimes it doesn't seem to have a temperature. At times it is a constant feeling – at times it throbs and the intensity goes up and down.

Pain is a problem for Saul. And it's a problem for those trying to help him. Saul has a reputation for being honest and a straight-shooter. When he says he feels something in his shoulder or in his arm people believe him. But they don't know what to believe is really going on – and that's because Saul doesn't know either.

Let's try to understand pain.

1st Attempt:

When someone says that their pain is killing them what we're hearing is a combination of two things: (1) they have a **hurt** and (2) they're **suffering** from that hurt.

On days when Saul feels on top of the world and he becomes aware of the feeling in his shoulder he probably doesn't suffer that much from the hurt.

On other days when Saul is feeling as though the bottom has dropped out of his world; when he's depressed or really tired; or anxious; the same degree of physical hurt might cause a lot more psychological suffering.

Did you see the pairing of words? **Physical - hurt** and **psychological - suffering**.

One part of the pain is physical and the other is psychological. (And both of these parts are real.)

One part is in the body (including the bones and organs and nerves and brain) and the other is in the thinking, emotional and biochemical systems that make up our psychology.

2nd Attempt:

Very often, pain is something that has a meaning for us.

There are many stories of soldiers who suffered physical damage to their bodies as a result of shell-fire but who lay quietly on the battlefield or in a field hospital, waiting for help.

And they knew that if they had suffered the same injuries 'back home' they would not have been able to endure it. Why the difference?

For many, the injury on the battlefield meant that they were now going to go home. They would soon be out of danger.

Some described the injury as being like a friend who had come to rescue them from the horror of war.

The **meaning of an injury** can determine the amount of pain we experience.

Picture little Johnny on the playground.

He is playing a game ("crack the whip") in which he is running with his mates and then is jerked so violently by the hand that he is sent sprawling onto the ground, maybe even scratching and bruising himself.

Within 5 seconds he is up and running after the group in order to "enjoy" the game again.

Now imagine that little Johnny's father gets weary of trying to get Johnny up off the floor from in front of the TV.

He grabs one of his son's hands and begins to pull him upwards.

Johnny is likely to scream, not only in protest but also in response to the pain he is feeling in his wrist or shoulder. In the first case, the meaning of the tug in the shoulder was that it was part of a game.

In the second case the same tug (likely actually less physical force on the arm and shoulder) was perceived as being a real injury.

The **meaning** of the injury or assault on the body can determine the amount of pain we experience.

3rd Attempt:

When I was going through my own chronic pain nothing made me angrier than to hear someone tell me, "Your pain is all in your head".

More than one physician hinted at this and many members of my family began to think this way, I'm sure.

No doubt some pain is the result of hysteria or other mental/emotional condition which creates a continuing experience of both hurt and suffering.

But a far more common situation arises when the body itself is the source not only of the original pain but also of conditions which keep the pain alive and well (if I can use such an expression).

It appears from new studies in the field of neuroscience that some pain perpetuates itself.

First, there is a path between some portion of the body which has been injured and the nervous system which carries pain messages to the brain.

Then there is a reaction from the nervous system back to the injury site; then there is a reaction from that site back to the nervous system, etc., etc.

It's called a feedback loop and some pain would appear to be the result of this loop. It's a **self-perpetuating pain**.

The loop is actually made up of chemicals which are released in the body's cells and nerves and once the loop gets established it uses the body's energy to keep firing so that we continually experience the pain.

I explained this to Saul one day and he came back with this:

> Oh, so it's like having your reflex tested by the doctor when he hits your knee with his little mallet.
>
> Only when your foot jerks up you hit him in the gut and he jerks forward with his mallet and hits your knee again and then….

Some have called these loops "reverberating circuits."

Doesn't much matter what you call them, the evidence seems to be that this is the reason some pain seems to take on a life of its own.

It goes on and on and on, with no apparent physical cause such as a lesion or rupture or inflammation to account for it.

Getting Pain Relief

The only instant pain relief that I am aware of is a shot of a powerful analgesic properly administered, directly to the pain site or to the nerves that carry pain messages from that site. If you've ever had "freezing" for a dental procedure then you know what this feels like.

Then there is the kind of pain relief which can be created through a narcotic which is administered intravenously through a needle inserted into your body (usually an arm). The pain relief may not be instantaneous and it wears off if the drug isn't administered in a high enough dose frequently enough.

Other than that, an anesthetic which puts you to sleep is a good way of relieving pain while it is being produced during an operation but something else may be necessary after you wake up.

But these are not the kinds of pain relief you need and they're not available through an book such as this.

You're looking for a way to reduce pain which you can use between shots of a drug or along with a drug or maybe instead of a drug. You're quite possibly suffering from long-term pain which doesn't go away even with prescribed medication and exercise or physiotherapy.

Now here's the bad news (first):

> *No one can guarantee permanent pain relief.*

This is true even in some cases when a surgical procedure (called a rhizotomy) is used to block or surgically cut the spinal nerves which carry pain messages to the brain. Why? I don't know. It may be that this is one of those situations where the pain is continuously produced by a local feedback loop.

Now here's the good news:

No one is always in constant pain.

Did I just lose you? Did you disagree at once and get ready to stop reading? Well, let me explain what I mean.

Even in the midst of excruciating pain there may be a moment, perhaps only a second, in which your attention to your pain might have wavered. Or, there may be a slight shift in the level of your pain. The shift may only be a slight decrease, or it might be a shift or change in the type of pain. For example, we might feel that our pain is a constant burning pain. Then, for just a moment, we might say that the burning changed to extreme stretching or to gnawing.

That's what I mean by saying that the pain isn't "constant". It can turn on or off, it can increase or decrease and it can change its nature or quality. It can also change its location.
We might start off saying we know exactly where the pain is and be able to put our finger right on the spot. Then, a few minutes later that spot might have shifted, however slightly.

Pain does these things whether you want it to or not. We're talking about very small changes; probably not large enough that you would be interested in them or think worth doing anything about.

But, the fact that the pain does shift means that the body energies (likely biochemical) are at work. And it is this shifting energy that we can tap into and consciously use for relief.

Here's more bad news (depending on how you look at it):

Pain relief takes work as well as time.

Not only can't you be guaranteed instant success at relieving your pain, but you're going to have to work at these methods to get any relief at all.

Now here's the motivational pitch:

Would you change jobs or move to a different city for a 1% increase in salary? What about 2%? I doubt it. *One or two percent is a very small amount.* Now bear with me for a couple of paragraphs.

Let's say you've been in pain for at least 6 months. In 6 months, if you had been awake all the time you might have been experiencing hurt and suffering for a total of 182 ½ days.

That's 4380 hours or 262,800 minutes. If you spent only 1% of the time working on reducing your pain that would be a total of 2,628 minutes – roughly 15 minutes per day. Two percent of the time would be a half-hour per day.

Can you invest somewhere between 15 and 30 minutes a day to relieve your pain or at least to reduce it?

Can you?   Will you?

You probably won't commit yourself to 15 minutes a day until you know what it is that you'll be doing. And this is fair enough.

What you will learn in the rest of this book are several skills which you can practice. They are skills which I have taught to children, to adults and to the very elderly. Not everyone learns all of the skills. Not everyone learns any particular skill to the same level.

Give yourself a fighting chance. Spend some time each day – or every-other-day – with these techniques.

Tell your partner or those around you that you need a little time to practice your pain relief techniques. Ask that you not be disturbed while you are learning. Share what you are doing with those who seem interested.

Understand that some people who care a great deal about you and your health may not believe that anything other than medication is going to be helpful for you. Thank them for their viewpoint and then practice the technique which you have chosen to work on.

Again, let me stress that you should consult with your physician or other health care providers about using any of these techniques. In 20 years of teaching people to help themselves to relieve their pain I have yet to come across a single physician who objected. In fact, the most common reaction which has been reported to me has been, "It can't hurt. Give it a try and let me know how you make out."

Caution: Do Not Remove *Necessary* Pain!

When is pain ever necessary?

When it is a signal of something which is badly damaged or out of balance within the body. The damage could be to a bone, a ligament or an internal organ.

The balance could be with the functioning of an organ such as the heart or liver; or it could be any one of hundreds of chemical balances.

Your physician or specialist frequently depends on knowing where you are experiencing pain and how severe the pain is. Knowing this can help to plan both immediate and long-term care.

If you use a technique to eliminate your pain **before it is properly assessed** you may be putting yourself at risk. Don't do it! Get your pain assessed first. Get as much competent, insightful, practiced diagnosis as you can and use the pain reduction methods which are then prescribed.

If, after using traditional approaches, your pain persists, talk over your options with your physician and bring one or more of the techniques in this book to his or her attention.

Ultimately, you are responsible for your own health but if you enter into a partnership with your physician or other specialist to share in your care then honor this. Be sure you have as much support as you can get from him or her and the rest of your health care team.

Mindfulness

I owe a great deal to the Buddhist scholar Shinzen Young, for creating a series of audio tapes and books describing a form of meditation called Mindfulness. He says in the preface to a recent book of his, that this method can be used to deal with actual pain but it is also useful for any situation in which people are experiencing bodily discomfort or dis-ease.

You may want to learn about mindfulness from his book which also comes with a CD: "Break Through Pain: a step-by-step mindfulness meditation program for transforming chronic and acute pain" (2004, Sounds True, Inc., Boulder, CO 80306) ISBN-1-59179-199-5.

As you will see from other chapters of this book, some pain relief can be achieved by using techniques which distract you or which take your mind off your pain in some way. Mindfulness does not operate on the principle that you should ignore your pain, or that you should deliberately try to block it out, or that you should run away or escape from it in some way. Mindfulness operates by running into the pain.

That's correct. **Mindfulness operates by running into the pain.**

It can take many years to become a true expert at mindfulness but here are the steps which I have used and which many of my clients have found helpful. Your particular physical pain may make some of these steps difficult or impossible but try to do whichever ones seem possible and appropriate.

- Let yourself be as physically relaxed as possible. Loosen any tight clothing, take your shoes off if that's possible, and take a few deep breaths.

- Identify the pain which you want to work on in this session. If there are several areas that are painful pick the one which is least bothersome and start with it. The others will benefit by having your discomfort reduced and your attention drawn away from them.

- Treat your pain as a source of information. It can "speak" to you in many ways. Start by identifying **the outline** of the pain. This is easiest to understand if you think of a burn to your skin.

- There may be a very large area which is in pain but at some point that area stops and beyond that you can sense unburned skin and lack of pain.

- Next, consider **the depth** of the pain. Is it a surface pain? Or does it extend downwards? And if so, how far? One-half inch? One inch? And is the depth constant or is it deeper in some places than in others? Imagine you are mapping the area of pain in the same way that the bottom of the ocean is mapped to show the undersea valleys and ridges; the plains and the mountains. You may even discover there is a specific place where there is a volcano or two.

- Consider **the volume** of your pain. That is, what is the space occupied by your pain. Is it flat like a pancake or round and long like a rolling pin or a salami ? Is it the same shape for its full length or its full depth ? Sometimes pains start out being very large and then taper quickly to a point. Others seem to bulge in the middle.

- Next, allow your mind to reconsider each of these features or qualities of your pain. Spend a minute (which can seem like a very long time) observing the outline of the pain. While you are doing this the depth and volume images might crowd in.

That's fine. Just return to the outline and focus on it as best you can.

- One of the things you may notice is that the outline doesn't stay fixed. It may begin to become blurry, or perhaps it becomes curved where it was straight, or maybe it forms very complicated swirls. Whatever happens, happens. There is no "correct" way to see the outline.

- (I have been using the word "see" in this exercise. Many people say that they can't actually see things in their mind. If you are one of these people you can still ask yourself "What do I sense the outline is like; and what do I sense the depth and volume to be?")

- After you have spent some time with the outline move on to the depth and then the volume. Try to isolate each of these features from the other two. It will take some practice but you will be able to do it.

- Now go back to the outline, then the volume and then the depth and cycle through these several times.

- After about 20 minutes of this exercise ask yourself whether your experience of pain has changed in *any* way. Perhaps, while you have been doing the exercise your attention drifted away and you were not conscious of the pain for a moment. That's fine and you might want to settle for this; but it's not the change we're looking for.

- We're looking for a change in the discomfort which you experience. The physical pain or hurt may remain the same, but learning how to isolate features of it can be the beginning of getting control over the feelings of suffering.

You might ask yourself, "What's going on here?" "How can thinking about or sensing or imagining the pain as though it were a real thing make any difference to how it feels?"

The answer is that when we focus our mind's energies on our experience we begin to separate all the things that make up that experience. We begin to separate the physical sensations, the meaning, the emotional impact and the perceptions we have of the pain.

Mindfulness lets us convert what we typically experience as a whole into its parts. And each of the parts is usually much more manageable and tolerable on its own.

You may have heard the expression, "The whole is greater than the sum of its parts." Think football or hockey or any team sport. Each player is a part but you need the parts working together as a whole in order to stop the other team and score points.

What mindfulness does is to reverse this. **"The parts are less than the whole."**

When you can isolate each part of your pain from each of the other parts then you can apply any one of several other techniques to deal with it. As you get control over each part, relief from the total is guaranteed.

Changing the Quality of the Pain

This technique can start with the one described as "Mindfulness". It can be added on to the results of the Mindfulness procedure or it can be used on its own.

The Mindfulness technique breaks the whole experience of pain into some of its parts. Just doing that will sometimes provide relief. But in a sense this is a passive way to deal with these parts.

The technique you'll learn in this chapter is a much more active one. In it, you'll not only take the pain experience apart but you'll change these parts.

The parts of pain that we'll be talking about are its qualities. We almost always know things because of their qualities.

We experience these qualities through touch, sight, sound, taste, temperature and we use terms such as rough, smooth, loud, sweet, hot, etc., to describe a particular object.

Here's an example. I'm thinking of an object which is of moderate height; has a round shape with two things sticking out the bottom and two out the side; has white hair and a white beard; makes a sound like "Ho! Ho! Ho!" and has a large smile on its face. (Hint: It's December 20th as I write this.)

We have learned which combination of qualities make up particular objects or experiences.

(Some people, using only numbers on three or four scales, can communicate what they are tasting or smelling to others who are also very skilled in detecting the qualities of smell and taste and who use similar numerical scales.)

And, while pain is not an object like a table or like a loaf of bread, it too can be thought of in terms of its qualities.

Here are some common words used to describe the qualities of pain: hot, burning, scalding, aching, piercing, white hot, shooting, sharp, deadening, throbbing, screaming, dull, and aching. And there are other qualities such as: bad, wretched, beastly, strong, and weak. And this list goes on and on as well.

This technique is based on the idea that if you can take your pain apart in terms of its qualities and then actively change these qualities in your mind then in many cases your experience of the pain will also change.

I must admit at the outset, that many people find this technique to be very strange. So strange in fact that they don't want to talk about it to their friends and family.

You don't have to.

No one knows what's going on inside your head and what you're saying to yourself. All they need to be told is you're learning to deaden your pain by using your powers of concentration. (You're creative. Think of something else if this doesn't fit for you.)

When I use this technique in my office or when I teach it I generally follow a script which I have recorded previously recorded.

- Sit or lie back and take a few deep breaths. As you exhale imagine a wave of relaxation that starts at the top of your head and flows gently down over your entire body. (Even if you are in severe pain or can't manage a deep breath you can likely imagine the wave.)

  (Repeat this three or four times.)

- Now let your attention move to your area of pain and if you are experiencing several different pains or types of pain simply pick one to focus on for the time being.

- Now become aware of the strength of the pain which you have chosen to work with. If you can, assign a number to the pain. Use a 1 – 10 scale where 1 is a very weak pain and 10 is the worst pain you can imagine experiencing. You'll come back to this rating later.

- As you continue to breathe as evenly as you can let your attention sink into the pain you have chosen. Become aware of the **outline** of the pain and imagine a line drawn around the pain that separates it from the rest of you.

- And as you continue think about the **surface** of the pain. If the pain were an object within you what kind of surface would it have? Would it be rough, or smooth? Would it be like a nail file or like a piece of silk? Just observe or be aware of the surface and its quality.

- Now let yourself become aware of the **temperature** of your pain. Is it warm? Hot? Cool? Is the temperature steady or does it seem to rise and fall, moment to moment as you pay attention to it?

- Again, just notice these qualities. You don't have to do anything about them and there is no right or wrong way that things should be.

- Let yourself really imagine the impossible at this point. Imagine your pain had a **flavor**. If it had a flavor, something you could actually taste, what would it taste like? Would it be sweet? Or sour? Or salty.

Perhaps it would be bitter, or taste like some particular spice: paprika, or cayenne, black pepper. Maybe none of these. Maybe you can't imagine a taste. That's fine.

Just allow yourself to keep as relaxed as possible. Keep breathing evenly and move on to the next step.

- If your pain had a **sound** what would it be? Would it be like a big bass drum? Or a flute? Perhaps a screechy violin or a thundering church organ. Maybe a jazz group comes to mind. Or a section of a symphonic orchestra.

- Now you've looked at or experienced the **outline, surface, temperature, flavor,** and **sound** of your pain. If you want to, take a moment to review these qualities.

- You might find they have changed and that you have a different answer now than you had a moment ago. Again, there's nothing fixed here. Nothing engraved in stone. Whatever happens, happens.

- Take just a second and go back to your 10-point rating scale and assign a rating to your pain as you experience it right now. Has it changed?

If it has gone up don't despair. Sometimes, thinking hard as you have about your pain might bring it front-and-centre. Then maybe you are more aware of how bad it is right now.

Take a break if you need to and then come back to this exercise when you're ready.

If the rating has gone down, you can be pleased with the result and just note that what you have been doing up to this point is something that you can do whenever you want to.

- Go back to the outline of your pain and see whether you can imagine changing it. If it is straight in some place can you make it curved? If it is jagged can you smooth it out?

  Push it in and pull it out. Pretend you are reshaping a lump of clay. See whether it resists or whether it can be coaxed into a different shape.

- Move on to the surface. If you found your pain to have a rough surface can you smooth it out? If it was like sand-paper can you change the grade of paper so that it has less grit?

If it was smooth like mercury or silk can you imagine it now having a texture like fabric?

- You might try to stretch the outline here and there; and you might try different surfaces on to see whether they stick to these new shapes.

- What's the temperature and can you heat it up (or cool it down)? Can you do both?

- Try to change the flavor to something you really like. Or imagine tasting the flavor in a very diluted form. If it was salty can you imagine making it sweet, or bitter, or sour?

- Is the sound of your pain high? Low? Loud? Soft? Pleasing? Displeasing? What can you imagine that sound becoming?

  How does it change as you simply experience it ? Perhaps there is no sound. Then consider IF your pain were a sound what kind of a sound would it be? And then change that sound.

- If you can, let your mind flip back and forth across these new qualities so that you have sense of what your pain could be now and contrast this with what you remember your pain was when you started this exercise.

- Ask yourself how your pain has changed? How do you experience it NOW? When you think about it do you feel that it has exactly the same qualities it did a few moments ago?

- And how strong is the pain NOW on your 10-point scale?

- Finish the exercise by returning to focus on your breath. Take three or four deep breaths, letting them out slowly and then try to sit or lie quietly for a few minutes.

Take this exercise slowly. You can repeat any portion of it as many times as you want.

Like many of the techniques you will learn this one can be used almost any time and any place; except, of course, when you're driving or operating machinery. Not a good idea to be drifting off at these times.

Turning the Volume Down

The more relaxed you can be in using this technique the better the results. So, you may want to use the techniques from one of the other chapters is this book such as Relaxation or Self-Hypnosis and then move into this new approach.

You are lying or sitting and you are aware of your pain. Or perhaps for a few minutes your pain has decreased. Or maybe your pain hasn't decreased but you are very relaxed or enjoying the benefits of some drug or medication and your pain doesn't bother you as much as it has at other times.

This is the perfect time to take control of your pain by changing how you experience its strength.

I will suggest a number of qualities of your pain. Some of them will be quite familiar to you, others may seem strange. Even if what is suggested here seems odd or even bizarre, play along with it. The objective is to help your mind to change how it experiences your hurt.

Begin by going into your pain.

What this means is, try to ignore everything in your inner and outer worlds except your pain. Turn all of your mind's energies towards your pain. Think of these energies as being like a very bright flashlight with a powerful, concentrated beam.

Examine your hurt:

- Is it a small clearly defined area of the body?

- Does it extend the full length of some limb?

- Is it deep within the body?

- Is it around or between the bones of a joint?

- Does it have a clear beginning and then spread or radiate outward from that?

As you focus on your pain can you imagine **how it would look** if it were an object? How bright would it be? If it's red, is it a bright, fire-engine red? Or flame red?

Imagine you have a control knob for this brightness and slowly turn it so that the brightness is decreased. The color can stay red but it can change to a dull red.

Perhaps the color is blue. Is it the bright electric blue of a bare light bulb? Or the blue of a welder's torch? Or the blinding bright blue of the sky when you first step outdoors on a summer day?

You can use your *brightness control* to dim the intensity or strength of this blue. You can imagine it being toned down, dulled; just as though you were looking at it through smoked glass.

And can you imagine **how your pain would sound** if it were a sound. Would it be the blaring of a trumpet? Or the wail of a siren? Or the beating of a huge gong?

Use your *sound control* to decrease the volume. Make it softer and easier to listen to. Don't attempt to change the sound itself, just its loudness. You might find the sound changes on its own as you concentrate on it. The trumpet may become a smaller sound on an organ; the siren may become a clarinet; the gong might become a low note on a piano.

There is no "have to" in this exercise. Anything that happens, happens. Whatever you experience, even if it's unexpected or strange is your mind's way of telling you that change is possible and that how you experience your hurt one moment may not be fixed for all time.

Perhaps you become aware of a buzzing or **vibration** that seems to be at the heart of your pain.

Use your *speed control* to change it. You may find slowing it down is easier than speeding it up but experiment with both. One of the changes may bring about a change in your pain to a more comfortable level.

"BUT", you may protest, "THIS IS IRRATIONAL!".

Yes, it is. But there is probably nothing to be gained by looking at the logic of how your mind processes your pain signals. There may be a great deal to be gained by suspending logic and focusing on your sensations.

If you do this, you can say you are operating on a **non-rational** level. Irrational suggests "wrong"; non-rational suggests "based on experience". And there is nothing right nor wrong about your experience. It just is.

Relaxation

One very common reaction to chronic pain is to become chronically stressed. And we know that stress releases various hormones and that these hormones can make pain feel worse.

So it becomes a vicious cycle: Pain > Stress > Pain > Stress, etc.

When we are in pain we can develop two kinds of stress: physical and emotional.

One typical kind of physical stress which we develop is called a bracing response. Think of it as the body's way of tensing the muscles to protect itself against further injury. We brace ourselves for the next blow.

This kind of bracing requires muscle tension and if we hold that tension long enough then pain can result. So we are into another cycle: $Pain_1$ > Tension > $Pain_2$.

Relaxation can work in two ways: I can relieve the muscle tension which creates one kind of pain and it can reduce stress which creates or increases pain in general.

Some people who are in chronic pain are afraid to relax voluntarily and they may seek the "benefits" of alcohol or drugs to do the job for them.

They argue that if they let their guard down (which is how they define relaxation) then their pain will overwhelm them.

They believe the time they have spent defending themselves against the pain will be wasted and that their defenses will crumble unless they continue to put energy into them.

I have found it very difficult to argue with clients who have these beliefs.

My logic and their logic don't seem to be on the same wave-length. In the end, I have had to say something like, "I want you to squeeze the muscles in your hands and your feet as tightly as you can and hold them that way until I tell you to stop." I then take a book off my desk and start to read.

Most people get annoyed after a minute or two and say they don't like my game and they release their tension.

My reply has been to say that there are whole areas of their body that are under the sort of stress they have just put their hands through but they're not aware of it.

I also argue that this sort of chronic stress is likely not causing their original pain but it is doing absolutely nothing to help relieve it.

At this point most clients see what I'm driving at and are willing to learn something about relaxation.

Here's the script I use to help people with general body relaxation.

Record it for later playback, or have someone read it to you while you follow the instructions, or read it through several times and then try the exercise. After you have heard or read the instructions three or four times you can likely do this on your own.

Progressive Relaxation

(I'm writing this section assuming you are able to move about freely and can select a place to sit or to lie down in order to practice the technique.

However, you may be confined in some way; perhaps to a wheel chair or to a bed. If so, make whatever adjustments you need to in the instructions so that you don't add any unnecessary stress to your body.)

- Find a comfortable spot to sit or to lie down. Loosen your clothing so that you do not feel restricted.

  You might want to undo a belt, or remove a tie, or remove your shoes.

- Take a few moments to become aware of how your body is supported by the chair or bed or couch you are on.

  Notice the spots where your weight is supported and the spots where you are not touching anything.

  From time to time check to be sure that you are as supported as possible. Use pillows to fill in the hollows of your back or under your knees.

- Let yourself sink into the chair or bed or couch. Feel the support.

- Take a few deep breaths and as you do so imagine that you are breathing in relaxation and exhaling stress.

  Imagine that the oxygen you are taking into your lungs is really like a gas that can reduce your bodily stress.

  With every breath you take feel the oxygen coming in and imagine the stress being sent out through your nose or mouth.

- Start now, by tensing the muscles in your feet. Clench your toes and hold this position to the count of 5. One...two...three...four...five.

Now release your toes as you exhale. Do this again and time your breathing so that as you release the tension in your toes you are also exhaling.

- Do this once more and notice whether you have tensed other muscles. Perhaps your calves.

  Try to isolate just the muscles in your feet. Try not to tense other muscles in your body until you need to.

- Now tense the muscles in your shins so that your toes are pulled up and pointing upwards toward your knees.

  Hold this position to the count of 5; keep breathing and try to time your breath so that you exhale on the count of 5. One…two…three…four…five.

  As you release your shin muscles feel the relaxation in them. Perhaps feel a warmth or a tingling. Do this again to the count of 5. One…two…three…four…five.

  Feel the relaxation as you release. And once again,
  one…two…three…four…five/exhale and be aware of how your muscles feel when you release them.

- Now push your toes out away from you so that you can feel the tensing in your

calves and hold this position for: one…
two… three… four… five/exhale.

Do this sequence again for: one… two…
three… four…five/exhale. And again:
one…two…three… four…five/exhale.

- Take a moment to lie or sit quietly and
  continue to breathe as evenly and deeply
  as is comfortable.

  Don't force your breath. Just let it come
  and go. Be aware of your chest as it rises
  and falls.

- Focus on your feet again but this time
  press your heels into the floor or the bed.

  This will put a strain on your thigh
  muscles and you may feel the tension up
  into your lower back.

  Don't do it so hard that you hurt yourself
  in any way. Just press down until you feel
  the thigh muscles tighten up and hold this
  for: one…two…
  three…four…five/exhale.

  Again: one…two…three…four…five/
  exhale. And a final time to the count of
  five:one…two…three.. four…five/exhale.

- Next, tighten the muscles in your seat –
  your "glutes". Tighten and hold for:
  one…two…three…four…five/exhale.

Be sure to keep breathing evenly as you tighten these muscles again to a count of five:
one...two...three...four...five/exhale.

And a final set: one... two... three... four... five/exhale.

- Next work on your belly muscles and perhaps some of the muscles in your lower chest as well. Tighten and hold: one...two...three... four...five/exhale.

  Again:
  one...two...three...four...five/exhale.

  And a third time: one... two... three... four... five /exhale.

- Shift to your hands now by clenching your fingers to make a fist.

  Try not to tense any other muscles in your arms; just your fingers against the palms of your hands.

  Hold it:
  one...two...three...four...five/exhale.

  And a second time: one... two... three... four... five/exhale.

  And a third and final time: one... two... three... four... five/exhale.

- Now draw your hands up and tighten your biceps so that your hands are pulled in tightly towards your shoulders.

  Pull in and hold: one… two… three… four… five/exhale. Another time: one…two… three… four… five/exhale.

- And a final time: one… two… three… four… five/exhale.

- Drop your hands back to your lap or beside you on your bed and take three slow breaths.

  Breathe in relaxation and breathe tension and stress out.

- Scrunch all the muscles of your face as hard as you can. Make it hideous. Hold it: one…two…three…four…five/exhale.

- Pull the muscles together again. Don't worry about what you look like from the outside and hold that face for: one…two…three… four…five/exhale.

  Now once more:
  one…two…three…four… five/exhale.

- Next, scrunch up your facial muscles one more time but this time, when you reach five release them very slowly so that you can actually feel the various sets of muscles letting go: The first set: one…two…three…four…five/exhale.

Now for a second time: one… two… three… four… five/exhale.

And a third time: one… two… three… four… five/exhale.

- And finally, lift your shoulders up towards your ears. Lift them as far up as you can and feel the muscles in your neck and upper back pulling. Hold: one…two…three…four…five/exhale.

- Hold again: one… two… three… four… five/exhale.

- And one more time: one… two… three… four… five/exhale.

- Lie or sit quietly for a minute or two and tune into all the sensations which you may be feeling in your body.

There may be changes in the temperature of some spots; different areas or muscles may tingle or feel quite heavy. Any response is fine.

If you notice an area that seems to want to tense up you can experiment by actually tensing it, taking a deep breath, holding the tension and then relaxing it as you exhale.

- Check your pain level now. Has it changed at all?

- Take a moment or two more before you get up.

  Make sure that you are aware of your surroundings and that you have something to steady yourself if you need it.

  See if you can keep any of the good feelings you have now and take them with you as you go about your next tasks of the day.

I have found that clients who are able to make the time to do this exercise twice a day, once in the morning and once in the evening before going to bed, report more restful sleep, less agitation during the day and frequently have a reduction in pain.

Self-Hypnosis

Self-hypnosis is a skill that many people can learn. Those who learn it best have had a one-on-one training session with a professional trained in hypnosis.

In other words, it works best to have a guide or coach with you who can help you to select the best way to put yourself into trance.

What I'm including in this exercise is a script which will help you to achieve a state somewhere between deep relaxation and sleep. Some call it a "hypnoidal" state.

You may fall asleep doing the exercise, you may not; and I have to admit that some people become irritated at the slow progression of the instructions.

If this is what you experience, STOP! You don't have to suffer in order to learn something that is meant to relieve your suffering! That would be crazy.

Can everyone be hypnotized? Let me answer this by asking you whether you have ever been a driver or a passenger in a car and as you moved down the highway suddenly found yourself wondering what happened to the last few seconds; or to the last mile(s) of highway?

Almost everyone has experienced this. It's called "highway hypnosis". You were conscious but somehow not really all there. You would probably have reacted to a dangerous situation if one arose.

Yes, this is a form of hypnosis that occurs naturally and so it's probably true to say everyone can be hypnotized to some degree.

The script that follows will help you to make changes in your reactions to the pain you experience.

I urge you to read or to record and then listen to this script several times so that you begin to anticipate or guess at what's coming next.

In this way you will be planting the expressions and the ideas of the script in your unconscious. Later, when you want to do the exercise without the script these thoughts and phrases will come back to you and guide your experience.

- Start by focusing on your pain. This may be difficult because you may be used to distracting yourself or to avoiding your pain.

- Focus on your pain and take a deep breath. Imagine that the air you are breathing in is flowing from your nostrils across the back of your throat and then to the center of your pain.

- Do this four more times. One.... two.... .three..... four.

- Now imagine you are going to visit a distant place. A place in which you will find comfort and peace. A place where there will be nothing to bother you and nothing to disturb you.

- To visit this place, imagine there is an escalator which runs downwards away from the place where you are standing or sitting. The escalator has wide steps and a strong handrail that you can hold onto so that you are very secure.

- You get on the escalator and you become aware that its movement is smooth and easy and you feel quite secure as it begins to take you downwards.

- You are breathing normally, easily and you are only conscious of your smooth downward motion.

- The escalator arrives at the first level down and you become aware that the entire area is filled with a warm red color and that there is a large arrow on a sign ahead of you.

  It points downward and you get off this first escalator and move slowly over to the second escalator which takes you and guides you downwards.

- The trip downwards is like the first one. Slow, smooth, secure and with a feeling of comfort and warmth. As you continue you become aware of the color orange which surrounds you.

  It is the kind of orange that you associate with peace and you can almost feel it on your face and hands.

- At the bottom of this escalator there is another arrow pointing downwards and you follow it to the next set of steps which move you closer to your goal.

  The color surrounding you now is a clear yellow and you let this color run all over you almost as though you were taking a shower; bathing in the glow of this color.

- This escalator moves you softly and comfortably and in the background you may hear some soft music. So soft.

- Perhaps the sound of a small piano, or distant organ; or maybe there are some voices humming.

- As you listen you hear other sounds which could be wind in the trees, or tall grasses being blown about. And there may be the sound of a bubbling stream.

These are just sounds. Coming and going, reminding you of places and times when you were feeling free and easy.

- Now you step off this escalator and on to the next. It carries you effortlessly and you are aware of a pure green color which fills your awareness.

  It may be the green of new grass or perhaps the green of the sea. It could be any green or all greens mixed together.

- You get off the escalator follow the arrow and find yourself surrounded by the clearest blue you have ever seen.

- You might recall some summer sky or a jewel. Or perhaps you saw that blue in a set of paints or in a picture. It is a blue that gently hugs you and makes you feel comfortable.

- And you continue with nothing to bother you and nothing to disturb you.

- Now you are at the last escalator which moves even more slowly than the others and gradually leads you down to the lowest level.

- On this level you are able to breathe evenly and deeply and to feel that there is a part of you which is so very, very relaxed.

And this part can drift. And it can look about or sense the peacefulness of this place.

- And you realize that this peacefulness is within you and that this place is somewhere you can reach whenever you want to.

  You can come here any time you want to by taking some deep breaths and remembering what this feels like.

- Or, you can take some deep breaths and get on an escalator and be guided here.

- You can stay here as long as you want to. And when you are ready to imagine leaving this place you can also imagine leaving some of your discomfort behind.

  When you return to the surface you will be feeling alert and refreshed and some of your discomfort, or perhaps all of it, will have been left behind.

- Now, to return to the surface take a deep breath and as you exhale imagine you are rising up from level 6 to level 5…and now up to level 4.

- Pause for a moment, take another deep breath and let yourself float up to 3… and then to 2… and finally at 1… you're back.

You're alert, feeling fine and ready to lay back and rest or to go on with whatever tasks need your attention.

What you will find is that practicing with this script several times will condition your unconscious so that you can enter trance more and more easily.

There are really two things to do: first, focus on something – it doesn't have to be your pain –while you take some deep breaths and second, have clearly in mind your intention of going into trace.

But don't force it.

Simply assume that trance will happen.

(Not necessarily 100% of the time but often enough that you will be able to use it as a reliable avenue to reduce your discomfort.)

Changing How the Pain Feels

Lee had the misfortune to be looking the wrong way when a cyclist cut in from the street across the sidewalk in order to make a delivery. When Lee got out of hospital several weeks later his hip had been reconstructed but he reported being in terrible pain.

Lee asked if I could use hypnosis to help him to cope with his pain. I used the self-hypnosis script contained in this book and Lee went home to practice putting himself into trance.

When he returned the next week Lee reported a strange discovery. My script ends by suggesting, "When you are ready to imagine leaving this place you can also imagine leaving some of your discomfort behind".

Lee imagined that the stabbing pain in his hip should be left behind and that it should become a dull ache rather than the sharp jabs he had been experiencing.

To his surprise, he began to experience his pain differently. He actually did leave the stabbing pain and it became a dull ache which he found much easier to cope with.

My research of the pain management literature has shown me many times that this simple technique can be very effective.

To use this approach it is not necessary to go into trance but it does work best if you can use the self-hypnosis techniques which I talk about in another chapter in this book. Once you are in trance, using this technique can be much easier.

Whether you use trance or not, one of the things that is needed is the _belief_ that you can change your experience.

How does this actually operate? Here's a description of the process in which a burning sensation is changed to something much more manageable. You can substitute your own experiences and use this as a model.

- Start by doing whatever you need to do to feel as comfortable as possible.

- Finish your immediate tasks and make sure you are not going to be interrupted for about 15 minutes.

- Spend a moment or two thinking about your pain as you are experiencing it right now.

It is likely that spending even two minutes focused on your pain will surprise you a little by showing you that it tends to change on a moment-to-moment basis.

It moves around a little; it gets bigger, then smaller; it gets more painful and then less painful, etc. None of these changes is large but it's interesting that what we generally regard as a constant pain is in reality one that shifts on its own.

- Try to find a word or a phrase that accurately describes the pain as you are experiencing it right now.

  We'll assume that the description is: "a white hot poker sticking into me."

- Now try to imagine a very small change in what you are describing.

  In this example, can you imagine that instead of a   poker sticking you it is a hot liquid that is pouring on the same spot?

- Keep at this until you find some other image which captures the original experience.

- See whether you can change this image (even if it is a small amount).

  Perhaps the hot liquid could be imagined to be coming out of a tap and that cool water could be added to it. Maybe the water could become extremely cold, almost freezing.

- Picture what happens to this new image as you continue to keep it in mind.

  The freezing could become numbing ("numbing cold"?).

- Compare your pain sensations now with the one you had when you started the exercise.

- Practice doing this until you discover a sequence of images that reflects changes in your sensations and see whether your pain begins to change as well.

Here are some sensations which you can experiment with:

Itching	Grinding
Warming	Pulling
Stretching	Rasping
Cooling	Trickling
Tearing	Prickly
Pressing	Burning
Tingling	Throbbing
Twisting	Squeezing
Numbing	Grating

The very first step will be to find some sensation that you can transfer your pain to. Another way of saying this is that you want to find a sensation that you can substitute for your pain.

Once you have that, the next steps are to find one or several other sensations that can be used as substitutes for one another. In that way your original pain can be made to be something else.

Then you may be able to move it into a neutral or even a positive sensation.

This is not an easy task but some people find that just the effort of trying to do it is distracting from their pain – a reward in itself.

Staying in the Here and Now: Thinking

We (my wife Susan and I) frequently say to our clients, "There is no future in the past". When we do so we're trying to have them realize that whatever happened in the past, their current job is to find a new and better way of living now and in the future.

Unfortunately, some people are so loyal to their past that they can't imagine having a different future. Change feels wrong to them. On the one hand they say they want to be without their pain; on the other hand, doing things differently and changing the way they feel is so foreign to them that they resist their own best efforts! Sounds bizarre? Maybe.

When you are alone, perhaps overwhelmed by your pain, or struggling to cope with it, the past has a nasty habit of intruding on your thinking. You begin to say to yourself, "Why did this happen to me?" and "It's been going on for so long. Enough already!" and "After all I've been through, and all the things I've tried, why haven't I got any relief."

There may be other times when you think about your future and find yourself thinking, "I don't know if I can stand this if it keeps going on this way" or "How much longer do I have to put up with this?" or "Why do I have to wait so long for the medication (or the specialists) to do their job" or "What does it mean that I will have to learn to live with it?"

We have heard all of these statements and many, many more like them over and over again as we try to help clients deal with chronic pain. You may have heard yourself saying these very words or perhaps you have your own versions.

What everyone who is in chronic pain tends to do is try to find an explanation from their past or something to blame from their past that is causing their current misery.

This is searching for explanations in the **there and then** – the past.

The other thing which appears to be natural is to wonder what the future has in store for us. Will things ever get better? This is searching for a promise in the **where and when** of the future.

Putting energy into these two quests is almost never helpful.

However, putting yourself precisely in the middle of the past and the future can frequently be extremely helpful. What's in the middle of the past and the future? The present – the **here and now**.

Here is a script which may help you to explore this technique:

- With your eyes closed become aware of what is going on in your mind.

- Do you hear voices? Are you talking to yourself? Are you hearing previous conversations?

- Attend to your breathing, make sure it is calm and regular and also continue to be aware or what thoughts, or sights or sounds you have in your mind.

- Some of these thoughts may be about the past. Some may be about the future. Whatever these thoughts are, that's fine. Just let them be.

- Just be aware of your thoughts, and images and whatever else is in your mind. See these images as though they were projected on a screen in front of you and hear the voices or sounds as though you were listening to them on headphones.

- Don't try to stop whatever is going on in your mind.

- If you find yourself being led off somewhere else other than where you are right now recognize that your mind is trying to go somewhere else and gently bring your focus back to the present. Stay with what's going on now.

- Check your breathing now and be sure to feel the rise and fall of your chest or your belly. Don't try to do anything special with this, just be aware of the breath coming in and going out of your body. And then return to your mind.

- When you find your mind drifting, be gentle with yourself. Don't judge yourself and say you're making a mistake by letting your mind wander off.

- The mind is built for wandering, for taking in information in the present and for wandering to the past and to the future.

- Practice returning your mind to the present.

- Your pain may want you to attend to it; to give it care or sympathy. Recognize this. Tend to your bodily needs if you need to or acknowledge your needs and make a contract with yourself to do what is needed as soon as you are through with this exercise.

- Be aware that you cannot make a mistake in doing this exercise. You will do what your mind and body need you to do.

- Practice at staying in the present makes it easier to do whenever you chose to. Some days it will be very easy. Other days will be harder. Practice will make more days feel easier.

- (You may want to use a timer and set it for 15 or 20 minutes to practice.)

- After you have finished this session ask yourself whether you experienced less pain while you were practicing. And ask yourself whether there is less pain now.

- Doing this exercise twice a day will be very helpful. Doing it more frequently will be even more helpful.

Staying in the Here and Now: Breathing

There is a variation on the previous technique which uses the breath as the focus of the mind. The purpose is the same as the exercise just described: to keep your mind in the present, in the here and now.

Here is a script which you will find easy to remember.

- You may do this exercise while you are sitting or standing. Or, if your condition allows it, you can do it while walking, running or exercising.

- Pay attention to your breathing without doing anything about it.

- Become aware of where you feel your breath. It may be in your chest, or your rib cage or perhaps your belly.

- Keep bringing your awareness back to these feelings in your body; the feelings that tell you that you are breathing.

- Your mind may wander away from your breath. That's natural and you can simply be aware of this and return your focus to your breath.

- Sometimes it is helpful to use a counting system to regulate your breathing and to provide a focus.

- Breathe in slowly and as deeply as is comfortable as you count silently to yourself: one…two…three and then hold the breath as you count four…five…six and then release the breath as you count seven…eight.

- You may find it is simpler to breathe in to a count of three and out to a count of three. This would go like this: breathe in, one…two…three,   breathe   out, four…five…six.

- You can experiment with different forms and rhythms. The purpose is to help you to focus on the act of breathing and to stop the internal chatter of your mind.

- When ideas suddenly appear that's normal and you can just let them drift off and return to focusing on your breathing.

- When the mind wanders note that it is wandering and then take control and return to your breathing. Don't judge yourself.

If focusing on your breath in order to stay in the here and now is too difficult – and it may be if you are having physical difficulties and pain associated with your breathing – you can use something mechanical as your focus.

A metronome that is set for about 60 ticks per minute works very well. Focusing on the tip of the second hand on a wall clock or on a wrist watch can also be used although this can produce eye strain and I wouldn't recommend it.

The bottom line: use something to capture your attention, not your imagination, and stay with it so that the past and future do not feel invited to the party. Staying in the moment, in the present, can have an amazing effect on the amount of hurt and suffering which are experienced.

The Eye-Roll Technique

Here is an incredibly simple exercise which can be used almost anywhere and anytime. The exceptions are, of course, when you're driving or operating equipment and as you will see, some social situations.

Here are the four steps of this exercise and you can do them whether you are seated or lying down:

- Sit or lie in as relaxed a posture as you can, keep your head still, look up as far as you can toward your eyebrows and as you continue to look upwards...

- Take a slow deep breath and hold it for a moment as you...

- Let your eyelids close, let your eyes relax behind your eyelids and exhale slowly.

- Now just sit and become aware of any changes you may be experiencing in your head, your mind, or your body.

The result of doing the first three of these steps may be that you move into a slightly altered state of consciousness. In fact, you may go into a slight trance.

(As I suggested, this is not the kind of exercise to do when you are out socially or sitting with a group of co-workers. People tend to get concerned when they see others rolling their eyes up as this exercise requires.)

What can you expect to experience? My clients have reported experiences ranging from "Nothing! Absolutely no effect!" to, "That was incredible! I felt as though I had just floated out of my body."

For most people there is at a minimum, a sense of calmness after exhaling. If you can simply keep your focus on your internal states – your mental and bodily sensations – you may find that you are able to dissociate somewhat from your pain.

By "dissociate" I mean drift away from, or feel yourself to be at a distance from, your pain.

Geoff, an accountant, suffered severe back spasms from time to time. He found that when he had a few moments of free time between clients, he was able to use the eye-roll technique to "space out".

He was fully aware of what was going on around him and yet was also able to enjoy a minute or two of stress reduction and calmness. At times, this was all that was needed to make the discomfort of the spasm much more bearable. There were even times when the spasm released.

Like the other techniques in this book, this exercise did not "cure" the problem. The spasms did not disappear but Geoff was able to obtain some relief by using this simple approach.

EMDR

If you have ordered this book through an internet connection (ebook) then you will be able to access the following link directly from this page.

http://www.emdr.com

It's the home page of the Eye Movement Desensitization and Reprocessing (EMDR) Institute, Inc.

EMDR is a controversial, but in my experience, highly effective technique for helping people to reduce many types of trauma. It involves an eight-stage protocol and should be administered by professionals who have completed a standardized training program approved by the EMDR Institute.

Mini-explanation

When EMDR was invented/created it involved having the client move his or her eyes back and forth, tracking the movements of the therapist's fingers which were held in front of the client's face. Through the years, other forms of signal have been used: tones, lights, tapping on the knees – almost any form of input to the client that involved stimulating first the left and then the right side of the body (bilateral stimulation).

During this process the client was engaged not only in attending to the bilateral stimulation but also to memories and feelings associated with whatever traumatic event they had come to deal with. This dual attention is believed to help the client's brain to process information about the trauma and to integrate it with feelings and beliefs about the trauma and the self.

EMDR and pain

One of the novel uses of EMDR has been to help people to deal with chronic pain. Sometimes pain can be clearly related to some traumatic event from the past (an accident; a rape; mugging; surgery, etc.). Sometimes there is no clear onset of the pain or no clear triggering event.

The standard EMDR protocol can be modified in a number of ways to help people to focus on their pain and on the feelings and beliefs which surround it. Sometimes it has been helpful to focus on a future state in which the pain is reduced or absent.

- **Self-help**: You might want to purchase a recorded program which uses a combination of imagery and tones in a way that simulates a one-on-one therapy session. It is called,

  "Pain Control, based on EMDR" by Mark Grant.

  He has also written a workbook which contains an excellent chapter (5) called, "EMDR: an information processing treatment for chronic pain".

  These are available through:

  www.emdrresources.com

- **Therapy**: You may wish to contact the EMDR Institute for the name of a qualified psychotherapist in your area who also has approved training in the use of EMDR.

  The EMDR Institute carries the following information on their home page and I heartily endorse their position:

  - EMDR should be administered only by licensed clinicians (or graduate students under supervision of a licensed clinician) specifically trained in EMDR.

- It is important that you take time to interview your prospective clinician.
- The clinician should have completed the basic training in EMDR (a two-part course).
- Choose a clinician who is experienced with EMDR and has a good success rate.
- Make certain that the clinician is comfortable in treating your particular problem.
- In addition, it is important that you feel a sense of trust and rapport with the clinician. Every treatment success is an interaction among clinician, client, and method.

In my own practice I have used EMDR as the basis for several approaches to pain relief and most clients have found these to be useful. Pain relief was achieved in the office for many clients who have then been able to continue to use the technique on their own or with the aid of a CD or tape.

A Note on Pain and Food

Marlene is in her early 30's. She is a theatrical director who is struggling to make it to New York where she believes fame and fortune are certain to be hers. She is the life of the party (nightly), she knows all the local bistros and she struggles with her weight on a daily, weekly and annual basis. She also has terrible posture as a result of early osteoporosis and complains to her closest friends and her therapist about her constant pain and the fact that she has sometimes contemplated suicide to escape from it.

When Marlene is out, which is always since she never cooks a meal for herself, she tends to eat a lot of pasta, to drink red wine and to order cheese plates for desert. She can linger over two or three strong cups of coffee and a brandy and smokes from the time she finishes her desert until she leaves for home.

What's wrong with this picture?

Here is a list of words that might or might not be related to one another. For some people, every one of the words in the left column can contribute to the conditions in the right column.

Alcohol	Chronic Pain
Nicotine	Over-weight
Pasta	Fatigue
Cheese	Stress
Caffeine	

Sometimes alcohol feels like the only way out. It offers an escape from the suffering although it seldom actually relieves the physical hurt.

What happens is that when people drink we become less and less aware of our environment – both internal and external. We begin to operate in a fog and although we can still be aware of our physical condition the pain tends to bother us less.

Smoking is interesting because it can lead to relaxation and this in turn can reduce the experience of pain. But on the other hand, it can agitate the body and many of the thousands of chemicals contained in smoke can act as irritants for unhealthy or damaged nerves and tissue. The same is true of caffeine in coffee.

Foods such as pasta, cheese and a host of other common foods such as chocolate, wheat products, meats (especially cold cuts) and eggs can increase some types of physical pain for some people. The lists of foods and the particular pains they affect are very long and complex. I am **not** saying do not eat any of the foods just mentioned. I **am** saying that checking out what you do eat against the type of pain which you experience is a simple and often very productive approach to relieving your pain.

If you are serious about finding possible causes for your pain, and this includes irritants which keep the pain above your ability to ignore it, then you owe it to yourself to consult a book such as:

"Foods that Fight Pain" by Neal Barnard, M.D. (1998) Random House.

One final thought: Foods can be irritants and make your pain worse but the right foods can also be soothing. The proper foods in the proper amounts can improve circulation, regulate hormones and the endocrine system and generally rebalance your system. It's worth a try.

Final Notes

Resistance

There is a form of massage called Rolfing. It is very deep and sometimes painful. The originator of this form of therapy, Ida Rolf, said that pain is just resistance to change.

There is a great hypnotherapist named Bill O'Hanlan, who had the same reaction I had we first heard this: outrage!

I had been pursuing a change in my physical condition and my pain for close to thirty years. How dare she say I was resisting change. Off with her head!

And yet, she was right in a way. What many of us do is to pick only those therapies and therapists that suit our expectations of how a cure for our pain should be brought about. If acupuncture sounds absurd to us we may never learn about it nor experience it. If changing our diet in particular ways seems too far removed from our back pain to ever help us then we may continue to eat the very foods that contribute to inflammation and pain.

Our failure to be open to the novel or the unexpected is a form of resistance. I don't believe that resistance is just another word for pain but I do believe we need to be experimental and responsible in our approach to our chronic pain.

Secondary Gains

One of the worst things someone in chronic pain can hear is that the pain is all in his or her head. The second-worst thing he or she can hear is, "They're just looking for attention."

In Psychology, the term "secondary gain" refers to a payoff or a reward which someone receives in addition to the goal which they are pursuing. So, I go to the doctor hoping to find an answer to my problem. Someone has to drive me to my appointment; people in the waiting room see me hobbling, bent over, as I make my way to the receptionist; she asks me how I'm doing and expresses her sympathy when I tell her.

The acts of caring which others devote to me (driving); the attention I get; the sympathy I receive, are all secondary gains.

I want my pain relieved – if that happened that would be my primary gain. All these other outcomes are secondary to that.

But, to tell someone or to suggest that their chronic pain is maintained or made worse by their attempt to get these secondary gains is not only disrespectful but, in my books, it borders on being abusive. It might happen on an unconscious level but this is a matter for a qualified psychotherapist to detect and discuss.

To be absolutely honest about this there *are* people who are malingerers. They fake the severity of their injuries or their illnesses. By doing so, they collect compensation and sympathy. No doubt about it, such frauds exist.

There are also many people who fail to pursue avenues of treatment because if they did get better they might lose the attention and contact they have with others.

These individuals pose real problems for the health system, and for health care providers

Nothing in this book will help members of either of these groups.

My hope is that for those who have been long-term sufferers there is some technique in this collection which seems to fit; that there is some description or script which seems as though it might be a way to support their healing process.

Information on the Web about Medical Approaches

If you, or someone you care for, is experiencing chronic pain and you want to know more about medications, and various medical treatments available you might want to go to the web site of The American Chronic Pain Association:

http://www.theacpa.org

The National Institute on Drug Abuse has a very interesting site which provides information on a wide variety of topics related to pain. It is searchable so you can likely find very specific information about the problems of concern to you:

http://www.drugabuse.gov/Infofacts

And here is a quote from the home page of a site maintained by the Ontario Consultants on Religious Tolerance.

"Everyone is aware of the extremely addictive properties of drugs such as morphine and heroin. But what is less known is that these drugs' addictive properties are primarily seen among healthy people who are not in pain. They become addicted when they use these drugs illegally for the feeling of euphoria that they generate. If a person who is in severe pain properly uses these narcotics for the relief of pain, they do not feel euphoria; they do not become addicted; they simply have relief from intense pain. A wide range of people are in need of such medication; they include individuals who are suffering from advanced cancer, untreatable back pain, and limb amputations."

Many pain patients are still being *under*-medicated because of their physicians' fears about creating addiction. If you are in that situation or someone you care for is in it – speak up! One does not need to suffer needlessly in order to heal from a wound.

Disclaimer

I need to end this book by repeating what was said at the beginning:

"This book is NOT intended as a substitute for competent health care such as that provided by licensed health care practitioners. The material provided is for information only and *the reader is strongly advised to consult with their own physician or health care practitioner prior to engaging in any action based on this information.*"

You may be discouraged with your progress using conventional treatments but please recognize that health care providers (your physician, chiropractor, physiotherapist, etc.) are constantly trying to find the right treatment for you. If it hasn't been found yet and you want to try one or more of the approaches outlined in this book talk to them about doing so.

Good luck and good health.

David Abbey, Ph.D.
Guelph, Ontario
2014